I0440112

Beginners Yoga

Flex Your Way To A Fitter ….. Trimmer you!!!

By

Natalie Johnson

DISCLAIMER

The content in this book is strictly opinionated and based on the author's experiences. You should seek the advice of a medical professional if you are looking to treat or cure a particular health problem or condition.

Table of Contents

Introduction

Thank you for purchasing the Beginners Yoga digital book. This will be your guide towards improving your strength and flexibility through the ancient exercise known as "Yoga." Chances are you have already heard the term used before, especially if you go to the gym because most gyms have yoga classes held in their facility. But for those who have never tried yoga before, it can look kind of odd. The common perception that laypeople have about yoga is that you have to bend your body in all sorts of weird positions and get uncomfortable. This is not the case for beginners. But as you progress, you will find those weird positions and postures to actually be very comfortable and relaxing to your body. But for someone who is out of shape, it may look too scary to try at first. Don't worry though because you are going to learn that there are all sorts of yoga techniques suitable for people of all shapes and sizes.

Yoga is more of a mental discipline than anything else. Sure we see it as a physical exercise where people are twisting and turning their bodies in unusual positions. However, these people are able to get into these flexible positions because their mind and body are now disciplined to do them. When you first try yoga, it will be hard to bend because your mind is telling your body to stop. So you will likely find it difficult and will get confused as to whether or not you are doing it right. Don't worry because nobody masters yoga on their first try. Just like nobody masters mediation, running or even lifting weights on their first try either. It takes months and years of practice before you can really advance in yoga. However, yoga itself is a never ending practice that you will keep working on for the rest of your life.

Contrary to popular belief, yoga is not an exercise performed by females only. Men often think this because they look at the yoga classes in the gym and see all women in them. But what they don't realize is that most gym classes of all types contain only women, whereas men are mostly in the weight room lifting weights. Gyms have unintentionally become segregated in that way, but they shouldn't be. Yoga is important to all people, whether you are male or female. Men just fear it more because they don't think they are as flexible as women. Although many women are more flexible, yoga can also cater to the strength qualities of men as well. This is something else you will learn about later on in this book.

Did you get scared off yet? Trust me yoga is not scary after you try it once. The hardest part is getting over the initial fear that is common when trying anything new for the first time. But after the first day of performing yoga, you will feel revitalized because you will have done things with your body that you have never done before. The body likes change, whether it is a change in movement or a change in your posture. Too many people these days get stuck in one particular pattern of movement or posture, which ends up hurting their back or cervical areas of the body. A great example of this is with computer use. People are developing poor posture in their backs and neck because they slouch over and stare at a computer screen for many hours each day. Yoga is the perfect way to correct this poor posture and get yourself feeling better again.

The book will first define what yoga is exactly and then go over the various types of yoga. There are physical and spiritual forms of yoga, which cater to both your mental and physical well being. Once you learn about them and the benefits they will have in your life, then you can learn about how to actually perform the postures and movements of yoga. Just remember to take it slow and not overdue it, especially if you are out of shape and have never done yoga before. Depending on your health status, you could end up hurting yourself if you twist your body the wrong way. That is why beginners are better off going to a group environment, like a gym class, to perform yoga and learn it. Then after you get more experienced and know your body can handle it, you can practice the poses and movements in the comfort of your own home.

Chapter 1
What is Yoga?

Yoga is often associated with exercises, but the true meaning of yoga is based on a disciplining philosophy created by the ancient Indians. The purpose of yoga is to enhance your body, mind and spirit to make you feel better and stay healthier. There are many religions that use yoga to get in touch with God or the spiritual world for accomplishing these tasks, such as Hinduism, Jainism, and Buddhism. However, yoga itself is not a religion. This is a common misconception in the west because people grow up seeing movies and television shows with Buddhist monks praying and flexing. So they automatically associate yoga with the religion of the monks without realizing yoga is just something they practice in the religion. Although yoga is a part of many religions, yoga itself is simply an exercise of the mind and body that can be practiced by anyone. You don't even have to believe in the spiritual world or God to benefit from yoga. As long as you perform the movements properly and clear your mind of all negative thinking, then you will be on the right path. There are various forms of yoga that focus on physical aspects more than mental aspects; and vice versa. You will learn about them as you read on in this book.

No one knows the exact date of yoga's creation, but researchers and scholars suspect it could have been over 5000 years ago. This era represents the beginning of human civilization, which was near the end of the Stone Age. There is only speculation as to which particular civilization or religion started yoga, but scholars believe it derived from Shamanism. This was the ancient tradition of healing by altering your mind to become one with the spiritual world. It was in this world that you could heal your body and mind. Modern day shamans use nuts, berries and edibles from nature to give patients this out of body experience, but 5000 years ago they only had meditation through yoga. Some say yoga was developed from meditation in order to heal the body and strengthen the muscles. Although yoga won't cure diseases or viruses in your system, it can heal the muscles when they are sore and make you feel better. 5000 years ago, yoga was the only medicine people had. Today it is more of a natural relaxant for people than anything else, but it still helps them become happier and lead more productive lives.

The ancient Indians developed six branches of yoga that covered all the physical and mental aspects of our lives. They are yoga of devotion (bhakti), yoga of the mind (jnana), yoga of selfless service (karma), yoga of self control (raja), yoga of rituals (tantra) and yoga of postures (hatha). Over the years, there have been variations to these forms of yoga made by different civilizations and religions. However, all the yoga types we have today were inspired by these six branches. In western society, the only one of the original branches of yoga that is still practiced is the yoga of postures, which is referred to as Hatha Yoga. This is the one you see in gyms all the time where people are getting into different postures and movements. The other five branches are mostly all mental based, which involve meditation practices and simply living your life a certain way that conforms to positivity in the mind.

Yoga Poses

Newcomers to yoga will probably think they will be stretching their bodies the whole time because that is how media has portrayed yoga for years. Even though stretching is involved in yoga, it is really about balancing all aspects of your body. Besides your mental and spiritual states, you need to develop your flexibility and strength. This is where the yoga poses come into play. Each specific posture in yoga will give you a specific physical benefit, which you will learn near the end of this book. Poses can be done quickly to generate heat from the body and burn calories. You can also do them slowly to help increase your stamina and align your posture towards perfection. Either way, you have to do the poses in sequence without stopping because that is how you challenge your mind and body. Remember that your mental discipline determines your ability to perform the physical poses as well.

Yoga Practice

Yoga is referred to as a practice more than an exercise. It is almost how a lawyer or a doctor calls their profession a practice. Yoga uses this word because a person is gaining more experience at yoga each time they do it. And since yoga is about enhancing your mind, body and spirit, which means you're gaining more experience at enhancing these as well. The same way a lawyer gains experience at their profession. The only difference is that anyone can practice yoga, whether you are a male, female, young, old, college graduate or high school graduate. You also don't have to be flexible or strong because these things will improve as you do yoga. After all, do you think weight lifters started out life strong? No way. They had to lift weights to build their muscles, just like you have to do yoga to build your strength and flexibility. The Yoga Practice will keep evolving for a person because they will keep getting better the more they do it. There is no point where you will totally master yoga because connecting your mind and body is a never ending process. Even the Buddhist monks who have done yoga for 50 years will continue to do it for the rest of their lives. Once you get started, you will too.

Yoga Classes

Yoga classes have already been mentioned a few times already, but it is important that you take them seriously in the beginning. I know you probably want to do everything yourself, and that is commendable. But the practice of yoga involves so many elements of yourself that you want to make sure you are doing it right. The yoga instructors who run yoga classes are experienced in many forms of yoga and will be your guide throughout your yoga session. They will instruct you on breathing, meditation, and chanting. These classes are great for practicing the physical aspect of yoga above all else. Usually, when someone is around a group of people doing the exact same thing then it makes them want to do it too. If you are by yourself at home then you have to motivate yourself to perform yoga, which is impossible for a beginner. This is the same reason why people who buy home fitness equipment never end up using it. They get too tempted to go back into the living room and watch television or go on the computer. In a gym, you are taken away from all these distractions and are motivated by the people around.

Chapter 2
Types of Yoga

It seems that yoga classes are everywhere these days. If you go to any gymnasium you are bound to see yoga classes held there. However, what these classes often don't mention is the type of yoga being taught. This is important because there are dozens of different types of yoga disciplines. Depending on your physical condition, health and experience, you need to choose the yoga that is right for your needs. Most gyms will offer free advice for members who wonder if they are suitable for their yoga classes. In a typical gym, the yoga classes are not too advanced. Gyms realize that many people who go to the gym are not yoga masters, so the instructors and personal trainers are very accommodating to the inexperience of their members. That is why yoga classes are great for beginners. Then after you get better at it, you may want to try other forms of yoga that are not traditionally taught in gyms. These are either taught in private yoga meet up groups or in religious circles, like a Buddhist dojo. But if you are somebody who just wants to experiment at home then that is fine too. Purchase a foam mat and put it in your living room or garage. Then perform any one of the beginner style yoga exercises mentioned below.

Physical Yoga

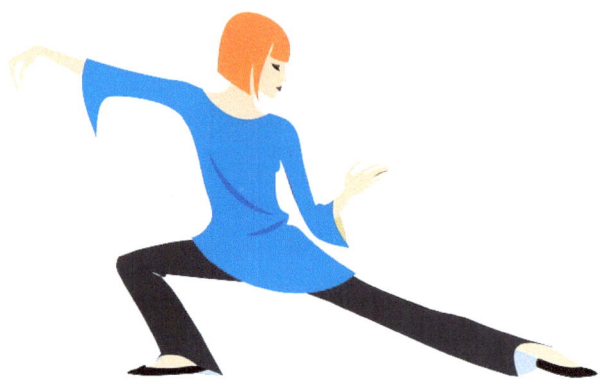

Anusara Yoga

Anusara is the most basic form of yoga that all newcomers should start out with, especially if they are nervous about trying it for the first time. In an Anusara Yoga session, students will get to pair up with partners who will help position their bodies into various twists and directions for them. This might sound easy to do alone, but if you are out of shape with no flexibility then you will want a partner to do this with you. This could involve lying down on a mat and simply trying to cross one leg over the other. Your yoga partner will gently push your leg across the other one. It won't necessarily hurt unless you have a former leg injury. If you don't then it will just help stretch the muscles in the legs to new areas they haven't gone before. Sometimes props are even used to help people focus their mind towards a particular direction.

Ashtanga Yoga

Ashtanga is a series of six strenuous poses performed in sequence. The idea is to move rapidly as you advanced from one pose to the next without stopping. As you move to each new pose, you will be inhaling and exhaling as you switch poses. The idea is that the breathing and the posing are linked together, which is known as vinyasa. This form of yoga comes from Mysore, India and was later brought to the United States in 1975 by Sri K. Pattabhi Jois. Many gyms across the United States that have yoga classes are likely performing some variation of Ashtanga. This yoga is great for people who want to lose weight because it is a nonstop yoga exercise where people don't even have time to catch their breath. This keeps the heart rate pumping faster just like a traditional cardiovascular exercise, like walking or jogging. Ashtanga is recommended for more experienced yoga students because of its faster pace. If you are a newcomer then try a slower yoga workout, like Anusara, before starting Ashtanga.

Bikram Yoga

Bikram Yoga is great for those who are looking to really sweat and burn off calories fast. This type of yoga is performed in a room with a hot temperature of about 105 degrees with around 40% humidity, such as a sauna room. While in the room, you will be performing a series of 26 different yoga postures twice in a row. The temperature will obviously make the posing a lot more challenging, both on your body and mind. This is great for athletes that want to build stamina because tolerating the heat while in motion is a perfect simulation to the high intensity you could feel playing sports outside under the sun.

There is an upside to Bikram Yoga. The heat will make you more flexible and loose, so if you couldn't touch your toes before then you might be able to during this yoga exercise. Just make sure you don't overstretch because that will lead to injury. Overall, this is a good form of yoga for anyone who is moderately in shape to those who are athletic. Newcomers might find the heat to be too difficult, especially if they are older and have breathing difficulties. Otherwise, try this yoga exercise out.

Hatha Yoga

Hatha Yoga comes from one of the six original branches of yoga developed by the ancient Indians. All of the modern yoga you see in gyms and meet up groups originated form Hatha Yoga. This simply uses a classic approach involving various postures and breathing exercises. More importantly, this is a type of yoga that is suitable for both beginners and experts. It is more of a stress relieving yoga exercise with many physical and mental benefits involving strength and discipline. Since it is meant for everybody, gyms are not afraid to put Hatha on their workout schedules. On a side note, Hatha is the only yoga of the original six yoga branches that is still used in gyms today. The other five branches are more likely to be found back in India, where it originated.

Kripalu Yoga

This form of yoga comes in three parts; getting to know your body, accepting your body and learning from your body. To get to know your body, you start out trying different poses to learn how your body responds to them. As you continue on, you start performing postures that you hold for a longer period of time along with meditation. After this, you sit down and let your body decide for itself what poses it wants to do. This is really a self empowerment discipline that teaches you what your body is truly capable of. By learning this, you can apply it to all aspects of your life.

Kripalu Yoga is great for newcomers to yoga that are trying to learn what they can do with their bodies and what they can't do. Between learning the mechanics and breath work of your body, you will get in touch with your spiritual side. Then you will realize that every physical gesture that you make is influenced by your mind. Kripalu Yoga helps you become more aware of that.

Spiritual Yoga

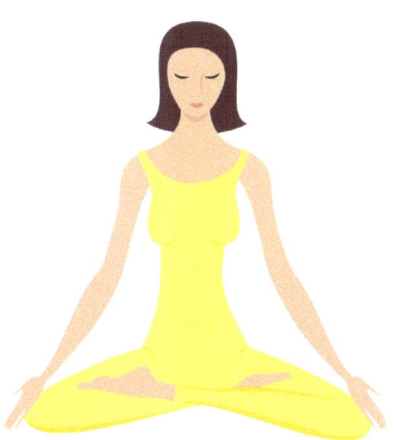

Karma Yoga

Karma is a word used a lot in Buddhism and Hinduism. Most people think it means that you will be punished in the future for the bad things you did in the past. At least, this is how western society views the meaning of the world. However, in the ancient religions karma referred specifically to your actions and where you would end up in the next life based upon those actions. This is what is known as the "path of service," which no one can escape from. With karma yoga, you come to realize that all of your experiences in the present are based on your past actions, whether in this life or a previous life. When you come to this realization through karma yoga, you are able to change your actions in the present so you are not bound to a future of selfishness and negativity. Basically, you can make the future better by taking better actions in the present that are selfless instead of selfish.

The great thing about karma yoga is that it is not like other forms of yoga where you have to physically exercise your body and get it all twisted up. Karma yoga can be done whenever we perform an action in our lives, whether it be going to work or helping your kids with their homework. It is simply a mental exercise based on the spiritual power of karma. But more importantly, it will make you a more positive person because you will feel good about your positive actions.

Tantra Yoga

Tantra Yoga is often perceived as a series of sexual rituals to experience what is sacred in life. Although sex is a part of tantra yoga, the rituals you perform go beyond just sex. Tantra practitioners are expected to experience devotion, humility, purity, cosmic love, contentment and truthfulness. Any action that gives you these experiences will be part of tantra yoga. For example, cosmic love is the love you feel for your wife or girlfriend. Then you experience this love with sexual pleasure. At the same time, staying faithful to your girlfriend allows you to experience devotion. If you two have a happy relationship, then you will have contentment. These are all things that make up the mindset of a tantra yoga practitioner. By practicing them yourself, you will find out what is truly sacred in your life.

Raja Yoga

Raja Yoga means "royal yoga." It is called that because it is considered by many to be the king of all yoga practices. The reason for this has to do with the fact that many of its practitioners belong to spiritual and religious orders. The exercises focus on contemplation and meditation. This is where you continuously stare in one direction without moving your eyes and clearing out your mind of all thoughts. You are only focusing on yourself and no one else, which is known as self mastery. It is through Raja yoga that one will gain respect for themselves so they can have more self confidence in their lives.

Jnana Yoga

Jnana Yoga helps people gain knowledge and wisdom in their minds. In other words, it helps you realize your true intelligence by surpassing the limitations you put on it in your mind. You basically perform this yoga by learning about the world and gaining true knowledge for yourself. Many religions, such as Hinduism, use the scriptures and holy text of God to gain this knowledge. For a modern day atheist, they will probably pick up a science book to get this knowledge instead.

Bhakti Yoga

Bhakti Yoga is the yoga of love and devotion. This is one that is greatly lacking the world, particularly in the west. People who practice Bhakti Yoga are able to see the beauty in everything and everyone around them. This creates love and acceptance in their minds as well as tolerance of others. This yoga is usually practiced by devoting your love to God and all his creations. By loving God, you love everyone else too.

Overview

You may be looking at all these forms of yoga and wondering which one you should do. The truth is they are all good in their own right. You just have to decide which disciplines are lacking in your body and mind. Remember that the yoga experience will be different for everybody. If you are too out of shape and scared to do the physical practices, then go for the spiritual ones. Sometimes we need to get our minds right before we can get our bodies right. Practice meditating at home and performing karma yoga in your life. This will be a good starting place for you to build up on because these two things will make you feel better quickly. Then as you begin feeling better, you will take more risks and eventually find yourself in a gym performing the physical yoga practices.

Chapter 3
Mental Benefits

When most people talk about yoga, they usually refer to their enhanced flexibility and decreased stiffness in their muscles. While these are great conditions to be in, the mental and psychological benefits are even better. You will be at peace in your mind with very few negative thoughts or stresses. With this mindset, you will be able to excel at many things in your life that you couldn't before because of your anxiety. This could be the ability to ask for a promotion, ask a girl out on a date or simply to motivate you to lose weight. Remember that if you have a healthy mind then you will be able to create a healthy body. This is an old saying that has always proven to be true. Think about all the people who are overweight or simply neglecting their health by abusing their body with drugs and alcohol. Their mind is so full of negativity that they use a stimulant to make their body feel better instead of focusing on their mind. Stimulants only provide temporary relief of anxiety, but then the side effects will make you feel worse in the long term. As for yoga, it is completely natural and only has positive side effects.

The British Psychological Society in the United Kingdom did a study on yoga. They determined that a person who concentrates on their breathing and how their body responds to various movements will be able to relieve stress. The reason that people in our society have become so overstressed and out of shape is because they only think about the stresses around them, such as their jobs, taking care of their families and so on. It eventually gets to a point where they are constantly stressed all the time without ever being able to relax, even at home. In a state like this, people can get angry for no reason and make everyone around them uncomfortable. The only chance someone will have is if they conquer these inner demons by being able to control their mind instead of allow their emotions control it. Yoga is the way to do this.

Stress and depression are pretty much linked together. If someone is stressed all the time then they are likely walking around frowning and not being very social. This makes sense because constant stress is like being in constant pain. Do you like talking to people when you are in pain? Of course not, and this is why yoga is so important because it helps relieve this pain. It does this by regulating the stress response system that exists in you. In general terms, yoga lowers your heart rate and blood pressure by helping to improve your respiration. It is from this that depression and anxiety will decrease. Best of all, you won't need expensive medications with dozens of side effects either.

Concentration

In our busy lifestyles, we tend to have multiple things on our minds at once. It can get so hectic in our heads that we won't be able to concentrate on what really matters or what we are doing in the present. For example, let's say you had an argument with your spouse before going to work. When you get to work you might be distracted from thinking about that argument, which will decrease your concentration from the work in front of you. Yoga would be perfect for a situation like this. It has been proven that yoga will enhance a person's concentration and memory in their heads by practicing the various exercises. Some people describe it as like getting rid of the static noise buildup in their brain and replacing it with muteness. That way they can focus their minds towards what they are concentrating on, whether it is the work at their job or a memory in the past they can remember.

Children

Mental stress relieve through yoga is not only for adults. In fact, it is even more crucial that teenagers and children get involved in yoga as well. Numerous studies have shown that adolescence is the time when a person develops mental health problems the most. This can often be seen in teenagers who are always acting angrily and spontaneously towards every situation that presents itself as a challenge. As a way to cope, their minds constantly wander into their thoughts and imaginations. And now with all the forms of media that kids get exposed to, like video games and movies, their minds are even more lost than they were before. If only these kids were brought up on yoga instead of MTV, they would become more well adjusted adults. Yoga, particularly Kripalu Yoga, has been known reduce and even prevent mental illness in children before they become teenagers or adults. There was a recently published study in the "Journal of Developmental and Behavioral Pediatrics" on students in physical education classes around the USA who got to perform Kripalu Yoga in class. In this type of yoga, you practice physical postures, relaxation techniques, breathing and meditation. After the study was concluded, it was found that students were in better moods and had lower levels of tension and anxiety. Most of all, they were able to control their anger which is something even adults have trouble doing. Since yoga poses no negative risks to teenagers, then it should be introduced to them in more schools around the world.

Post Traumatic Stress Disorder

Beyond all of the ordinary stresses and everyday mental battles that people deal with, one of the hardest battles has to do with traumatic experiences. People who have served in the military and gone to war suffer from deep depression, sadness, anxiety, stress and lack of concentration. All they can think about are the horrible memories of war. Their dreams will be filled with nightmares and constant flashbacks of their traumatic experiences. This is what is known as post traumatic stress disorder, or PTSD. However, it is not only military veterans who suffer from this disorder. Anyone who has been through any type of traumatic experience will have this, such as rape victims, policemen, prisoners, or anyone else who experienced something horrific.

The solution that society has for these people is to give antidepressants to them or various other prescription medications that alter their mental state. But like drugs and alcohol, medication only has temporary effects before they become habit forming and causing additional side effects that nobody wants. Therefore, yoga is the only healthy treatment left for people who suffer from PTSD. The American Psychological Association has seen Hatha Yoga reducing the symptoms of PTSD in patients. It is not a cure because there are no cures for PTSD. But yoga will certainly help people control their thoughts and not let them drift towards the negative thoughts and flashbacks of their traumatic experience.

Instead, they can direct their thoughts towards things they have in their present life, such as family, friends and career.

Chapter 4
Flexibility Benefits

Yoga utilizes flexibility a lot in its practice. People often think that this part of yoga is just for show. They don't realize that flexibility helps reduce your stress levels and simply improves your overall health. You don't have to do yoga for hours every day to get these benefits either. If you were to just devote 15 minutes a day to any physical form of yoga then your body would burn more calories, increase its blood flow throughout the body and improve your mental discipline. All of these benefits have been placed into five categories that truly show why the flexibility side of yoga is important.

Less Chance of Injury

Whether you are an athlete or not, you probably remember in grade school when your gym teacher told you to stretch out before running the mile on the track. They didn't tell you that just to give you something extra to do. Stretching is a form of flexibility, which will improve your physical performance in any exercise that you do afterwards. Not only that, but it will improve your range of motion by making your joints more flexible. Since this makes it easier for your body to make the movements, you won't need as much energy to sustain them. This means you will be more coordinated when doing any physical exercise, like running, and you will less likely fall down or get injured in some way from poor movement.

Better Posture

Yoga movements basically consist of a series of postures that force you to stretch and bend while holding that position. You perform the movements gradually as you utilize the muscle's full range of motion. Each time you get into a new position, you hold it for about 20-30 seconds. You take the positions as far as you can go in this manor without feeling pain. Research studies have shown that yoga stretching will reduce soreness in the muscles and improve your muscular balance. Once you have balance in the muscles, your posture will be improved.

Treat Lower Back Pain

Older people with bad backs are often told to go to yoga classes because it will help with their lower back pains. Of course, younger people can also risk injury to their lower backs, especially if they lift heavy objects or weights. But even if you don't lift heavy objects, the muscles contract a lot throughout the day, regardless of whether you are sitting or walking. Either way, your muscles will become stressed just by using them normally for long periods of time. That is why people who sit in a chair for 8 hours per day will eventually stand up and hold their lower back because all the sitting and poor posture caused it pain. Therefore, everybody should practice yoga for this reason. The stretching that is performed during yoga will relax the muscles in the back and reduce the sensation of lower back pain that one may be feeling frequently.

Soft Tissues Receive More Nutrients and Blood Flow

When you stretch your muscles with yoga you are increasing the blood flow to the muscle tissues. While the blood flow increases, essential nutrients are being delivered throughout the body. This also increases the synovial fluid in your joints, which is the lubricant in the joints that helps transport nutrients to it from the body. After this happens you will have less joint pain and a greater range of motion. More importantly, you will have a lesser chance of having joint degeneration as you get older.

Improve Your Overall Health

All of the benefits of flexing we have talked about so far, such as better posture, more nutrients in the blood stream, reduced risk of injury and so on, are all things that will improve your overall vitality and health. After you have been practicing your flexing with yoga, you will notice less soreness in your muscles, better overall movement with your body and a better physical performance during exercises. More importantly, your stress levels will go down and your mood will improve. After all, when we are stressed our muscles tend to get tight, which makes moving and breathing rather difficult. By using yoga to relax the muscles, you will breathe better and move better in the process. This is how yoga works the mind, body and spirit all in one shot. Just make sure you regularly perform yoga with a flexibility routine at least a few times per week. Then once you get better at flexing, try to challenge yourself by doing them faster in a sequence and with more moves.

Chapter 5
Strength Benefits

Yoga is often associated with flexibility and endurance because of the sequential posing and flexing of the body. What people don't realize is that a person's strength is also increased from doing yoga. Many of the yoga movements involve resistance training, which is where you push and pull the weight of your body to support the posture of the movement. Anytime you push up from the floor, for example, you are pushing the weight of your body. This is why pushups are almost like doing bench presses because both exercises work your pectorals, or chest muscles. The only difference is pushups do not require a barbell with weight plates. It only requires you to push your own body weight up from the floor. Resistance training in yoga is very similar to this concept, except that you hold the poses and weight of your body in place. This is what is known as isometric strength training, which is when you strengthen your muscles without moving your body or joints. In the weight room, this would be like if you lifted a heavy barbell up in the air and just left it there for a minute. Instead of pushing the weight up and down repeatedly, you hold it in the air to perform an isometric exercise. Yoga is just like this except you don't use any third party weights. You just train your body through isometric poses.

Strength Training & Yoga Combination

If you are serious about getting big muscles then you will need to do strength training and yoga together. Even though yoga will strengthen your muscles, you will never be able to lift super heavy weight with just yoga alone. However, by performing yoga with the strength training you will be able to increase the endurance of your workouts and be less prone to injury while lifting heavier weights. After all, yoga will make it so your joints are more flexible and trained to sustain the resistance of heavy weight. You just need to learn a few methods to do strength training and yoga together in the same week. Here are two of the best methods for doing this. Many people do method number one only because it involves high intensity and limited yoga workouts. Method number two focuses more on the yoga and limits the intensity of strength training; however, this is only a temporary method.

Method # 1)
If you are actively lifting weights and are trying to get into yoga, wait until you approach your recovery day. This is the day you would have normally taken off to let your muscles repair themselves. But now instead of taking it off, devote this day to one full yoga workout session. Then when you go back to your weight lifting days, do a 15 minute yoga session after your normal weight workout. Choose 3 or 4 poses to work on during these 15 minute yoga sessions. Switch the poses on every following day so you learn new ones. Then go back to the old ones during the next week and repeat the process.

Method # 2)
For those who truly want to focus on their yoga, you will need to do more yoga sessions than weight lifting workouts. In other words, you should reduce the intensity of your strength training for about 12 weeks while you incorporate yoga into the mix. In fact, devote about 2 days per week to strength training with weights. Do not lift heavy weights during this time. Just treat

these initial days as "light weight" days. Then on four other days you will do full yoga workout sessions that last at least an hour each. Try to get 10 poses into these sessions with more intensity and hold the poses for longer periods of time. For best results, join a yoga class at your gym so that an instructor can motivate you to move faster. Then on the last day, you will do both strength training and yoga in the same day. After doing this routine for twelve weeks straight with no rest days for anything, go back to the previous method in this list and increase the intensity of your strength training workouts once again. Just remember to do your 15 minute yoga sessions after these workouts.

Why Yoga Isometrics Strengthen Muscles

You may still be confused as to exactly how static weight lifting or yoga poses can help strengthen your muscles. These isometric exercises cause your muscles to get tense while holding the contractions. What happens during this process is the blood flow to the tense muscle gets reduced while the muscle tissue grows longer. The longer you hold these muscle contractions the bigger your muscles will get. So if you are looking to increase the size of your muscles then hold your yoga poses or isometric exercises for as long as possible. If you are a woman simply looking to tone up then you can experiment with set time limits of 30 seconds to a minute of holding a particular pose.

Yoga Isometrics and Aging Muscles

As people age, their muscle tissue begins to shrink. This means their muscles are not as big as they once were during their youth. This age related muscle loss starts for most people in their early 30s and picks up more around their 40s. But they lose more than just their youthful and toned muscular appearance. They also start having joint stability and motion problems as well. This weakens their sense of balance and stability, which then limits their ability to do the normal everyday activities that they are used to doing. What happens is the body stops producing as many hormones as it used to in order to help your muscles grow. Not only that, but an older person will have more trouble digesting essential amino acids that are responsible for repair muscles after a workout.

Isometrics are a counter balance to these disastrous things that occur inside our bodies as we become older. Now you won't be able to completely stop muscle loss, but you can at least reduce its decline by stabilizing its growth with yoga isometric poses. Then if you add strength training workouts on top of these sessions, it will reduce muscle decline even more. Basically, you just have to work harder when you get older in order to keep your muscle growth. It might not sound nice, but that is the brutality of Mother Nature.

Take Caution

No matter what exercise you do, your blood pressure is bound to increase from it. What you may not realize is that isometric exercises cause your blood pressure to rise the most. After all, when the muscles contract they force blood out of their tissue, which then ends up in your blood stream. This is how you get increased blood pressure. Even something as simple as holding your breath will cause you to have a blood pressure increase. Since yoga utilizes both breathing and isometric exercise techniques, this means you will be causing a rapid boost to your blood pressure. So if you suffer from any existing high blood pressure conditions or have a high risk of stroke, then you may want to consult your doctor before trying yoga.

Also take note that isometric exercises don't strengthen the entire muscle that is being worked. The reason is because your muscles are not moving or changing length while the isometric exercise is being performed. That means the only area of your muscle that will gain strength is a small 20 degree area around the joint angle that is being held during contraction. Of course, you can perform multiple isometric exercises that hit different angles during your yoga workout. That way you hit other areas of the muscle that didn't get strengthened before. For example, let's say you do a pushup pose on the ground to work your chest muscles. In order to work different parts of your chest, you would change the position of your hands during each pose. During the first pose, you would position your hands wide out past your shoulders. Then on the next pose you would position them at shoulder length and on the final pose they would go inward near your chest. Also, the depth of your pushup can change with each pose as well. One pose could have your body being held all the way up, the next pose you hold your body up half way and the final pose you hold your body up a little bit off the ground. Mix these with the variety of hand positions and you will work every part of your pectorals with merely isometric exercises. This same philosophy can be applied to all yoga movements and postures. Just keep changing your positions around to work all angles of the muscle. Even if you are doing strength training in the weight room, you will still want to do yoga isometrics on all angles of your muscles. That way you don't have just one angle that is stronger than the other angles.

Chapter 6
Beginners Workout Poses

In this chapter we will go over the basics of completing a yoga workout. Do not let the word "workout" confuse you though. We are not just talking about physical exercise. Yoga is an exploration of the mind and body. It is only a workout because you will be sweating while performing different exercises and poses.

You already know there are many variations of yoga which all have their own concepts and purposes. However, many of these variations use similar posture techniques, but just in different ways. Here you will be able to prepare yourself for some of these basic techniques, so that you can mentally know what you are getting yourself into. Don't worry you won't be twisting your legs around your head on the first day. Just relax and process the information slowly. The techniques may look hard, but with a little practice you will get good at them in no time.

Your First Pose

The first pose you do will be the easiest. This is just to warm up your body and get it motivated to start. What you will do is get in a seated position on the floor. Make sure you are comfortable; sit on a mat or light cushion if necessary. Keep your back and head straight as you sit on the floor. This position will lengthen your spine, open the hips and simply set your mind at peace. Then you cross your legs in a lotus position like you were taught in grade school, also called "Indian Sitting." However, this time when you cross your legs you will be putting your feet directly underneath your knees. Then rest your hands with the palms up on top of your knees.

Now comes the part that gets tricky. You will press your hip bones towards the floor and drop down your shoulders and back while sticking your chest towards the front. Next you relax your belly, jaw and face. Place your tongue on the roof of your mouth and let it rest there. Breathe in deeply through your nose and feel the air go down into your belly. Once it is there, hold it there for as long as possible.

The Downward Facing Dog Pose
If you feel that you have gotten good at the first pose, then you can try one a little more advanced. This is the downward facing dog pose, which might sound strange but it is actually a very well recognized pose. Basically, it is a stretch that rejuvenates the body, strengthens the arm muscles and calms depression in the mind.

To perform this pose, you first get on the floor with your hands and knees. Position your hands just slightly away from your shoulders and your knees below the hips. Spread your fingers in each hand and turn your hands slightly outward. Let out a nice gentle breath and begin to lift your knees up off the floor while keeping the other body parts in the same position. The knees can be slightly bent at first. Then lift the heels of your feet away from the floor, but keep your toes on the floor. You will want your toes and hands to be the only two body parts touching the floor. The rest of your body will be extended into the air as far as possible. In other words, your buttocks should be the highest point in the air while in this position. Hold it for 30 seconds. To challenge yourself more, try extending your hands farther out and then hold that position. You will find that the farther your hands are from your feet the harder it will be. Keep challenging yourself like this until you find it impossible to hold for 30 seconds.

Mountain Pose

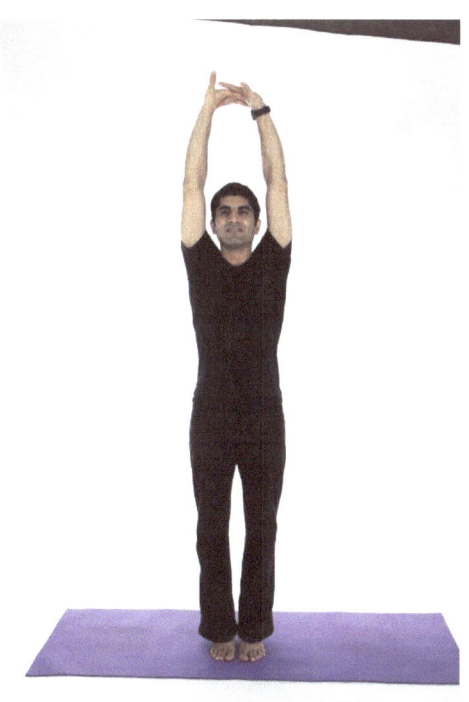

The mountain pose is the easiest yoga pose. It is also considered to be the foundation of all yoga poses. Anybody with the ability to stand on their two feet and raise their arms in the air can do this pose. This is basically all you do. You stand straight and tall with your feet together. You relax your shoulders with your arms by your side. Take a deep breath and then slowly raise your hands above your head until your palms touch each other. Keep your arms straight while doing this. Try to reach up as high as you can as if you were reaching for the sky. What this pose will do is straighten your posture when practiced regularly, which will result in reduced back pain. In addition, it will strengthen your ankles, knees, thighs, buttocks and abdomen.

The Warrior Pose

There are many variations to this pose, but we will discuss the most common variation. Basically you stand with your legs at least 3 feet apart. One foot is stretched far in back of you while standing and the other food stays in front of you. Next you extend your arms straight out at shoulder level with your palms facing down. Try to bend the leg in front of you to a 90 degree angle and keep it positioned just above your ankle. Keep this pose for one minute, then switch legs and do it again. This pose will strengthen the flexibility in your legs and hips. It will also reduce soreness in your leg muscles.

The Tree Pose   The tree pose is a more advanced version of the mountain pose. This is where you stand straight and put your feet together, and then raise your arms straight up into the air as far as they will go. However, this time you will lift your right leg and place the bottom of your right foot onto the inside of your left thigh. All of this is done while standing and holding the other body parts in position. So basically, you will end up standing on one leg with your arms straight up into the air. This requires a lot of balance and won't be easy for people who haven't perfected their yoga poses yet. Either way, you probably won't keep perfect balance during the tree pose at first because standing on one leg might be new to you. But don't worry because the more you practice the more you will get better and learn to keep perfect balance. This balance is what all yoga practitioners want to achieve because it will help them move better and perform better in other workout routines.

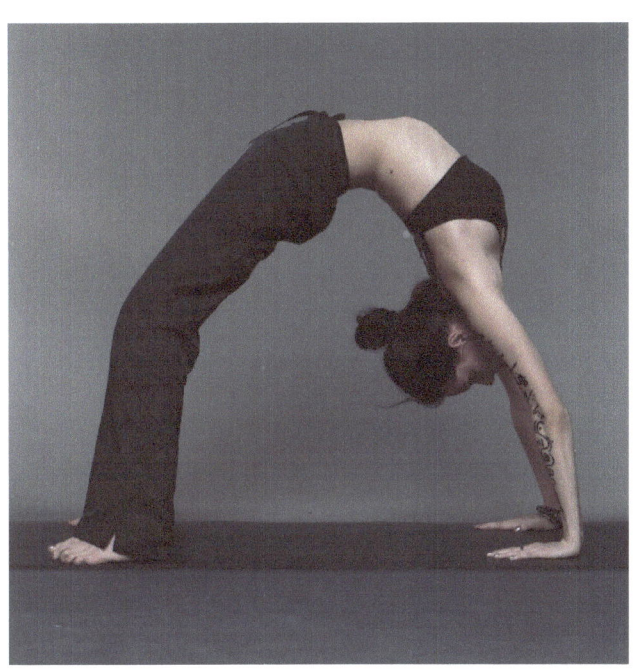

Bridge Pose

The bridge pose is a moderately difficult exercise, but not too hard. It strengthens your chest, spine, hips and neck as well as your buttocks, hamstrings and back muscles. More importantly, it reduces stress levels and greatly improves blood circulation throughout the body. You first lie down on the floor with a mat under you. Next you lift your pelvis off the floor and extend it as high as it will go. To do this successfully, you will want to position your legs to where your knees are directly above your feet. Then place your arms by your sides with palms facing down. Exhale slowly and push the heels of your feet against the floor to lift your hips up into the air. While your hips are in the air, try to clasp your hands together underneath your lower back. Keep your arms pressed down on the floor and as straight as possible. Try to bring your chest as close to your chin as you can. Hold this exact position for one minute. Now if you find this pose to be difficult or if you are unable to hold it for one minute, you might not be ready for it yet. What you can do is place a pillow underneath your tailbone, so that it will help you keep your pelvis in the air in case you keep falling down during the pose. Think of the pillow as the "training wheels" of the bridge pose. Eventually, you will get more experienced and won't need the pillow anymore.

The Pigeon Pose

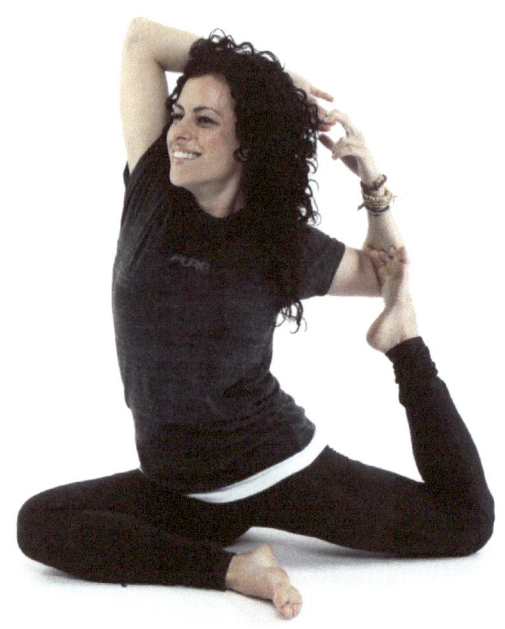

If you are looking for a pose that helps lower back pain by strengthening the back muscles, the pigeon pose is what you want to do. First place a mat on the ground and sit on it. Extend your right leg straight in back of your body and cross your left leg over to the right side. Try to make your right leg go as far back as it can. Now straighten out the posture in your torso by keeping your shoulders up in the air. Hold this position for 15-30 seconds and then switch legs. So now your left leg is extended in back of your body and your right leg is crossed over to the left. Do this for 15-30 seconds and repeat a couple more times. Eventually, you will be able to go longer and later incorporate it into other yoga sequences.

Shoelace Pose

The shoelace pose is what you would normally do after a yoga session. It is a recovery pose that works especially well after you've done exercises with lots of hip hinging movements. It also stretches the gluteus muscles in your buttocks to give them extra strength as well. You first place a mat on the floor and then sit on it. Then cross your right leg over your left leg and make the left leg cross underneath the right leg. Both legs will basically be crossing each other as far as possible. This is like making a shoelace out of your legs because you are tying them like a knot. It is okay if you have to hold the top leg to keep it crossed over the bottom leg. While you are doing this, keep your back and neck as straight as possible. Hold this position for 30 seconds and switch the legs. So this time your left leg is crossed on top and your right leg crosses on the bottom.

Reclined Spinal Twist

The reclined spinal twist will release the toxins and tension from the organs of your body, and calm the central nervous system in the process. All the twisting that is done in this pose will be like wringing out your organs like a wet sponge. But instead of water dripping out, the toxins and free radicals will be wrung out instead. This results in your organs being detoxified and stimulated. Yoga instructors often tell their students to squeeze out the tension and anxiety in their body while performing this pose. The harder they squeeze the more relief they feel.

To perform this pose, place a mat on the floor and then lie your back down on it. If you want to you can rest your head on a pillow or soft blanket to support your neck. Leave your arms down on your sides and let them rest there for now. Bring your knees up to your chest and hold them there with your hands. Release your left leg and extend it straight on the floor while still holding your right knee to your chest. Now extend your right arm straight out onto the floor at the same level as your shoulders. You will then be shifting your hips to the right while keeping your left hand on your right knee. Exhale slowly, and move your right knee to the left side of your body. Make sure your left hand is still holding your right knee, but only gently. Turn your head to the right side of your body and away from the direction of your right knee. Extend your knee over as far as it can go without forcing it with your hands. All of the tension should be in your hips and legs. Hold this pose for about 20 breaths and then do the pose again using the opposite legs and knees.

The reclined spinal twist is definitely recommended more for experienced yoga practitioners. You need to already be flexible and have no preexisting joint problems. For anyone who is older and sufferings from osteoporosis or some other joint condition, ask a doctor before performing this yoga pose.

Conclusion

Congratulations. You made it all the way to the end of the book. Hopefully by now, you have a good understanding of yoga and how it can be beneficial to your life. The common perception of yoga is so misleading amongst the general public, which is why I wrote this book. I wanted to educate people on what yoga really is all about and how it is different than simply flexing or doing weird looking poses. Yoga is a practice that enhances a person's body, mind and spirit. These are the three elements that make up who we are and how we behave. If you just work on one or two of these elements then the others will be neglected, which will eventually cause you to become a person that you don't want to be. For example, if you just lift weights everyday to relieve stress, then it will only cause temporary relief of that stress. Eventually, your mind and spirit will still be filled with negativity and uncertainty about life. Remember that yoga makes you discover who you really are inside as well as outside. You will discover how far you can push your body and then have a spirit that is determined to enhance itself. This is done through physical movements, postures and meditation of the mind. After reading this book, you now know how to do all of these things.

Yoga is a practice that can be performed by anybody. If you tell people you know that you want to try doing yoga, they may laugh or think you are going to become a Buddhist monk. These are very bad stereotypes that do not represent the true meaning of yoga in anyway. People who criticize you for trying out yoga simply do not understand it. They don't realize yoga is not a religion nor is it an exercise. It is a practice that balances your body, spirit and mind. As you learned, there are physical and mental yoga types that cater to your mind, body and spirit. Some people may perform physical yoga more than mental yoga; and vice versa. The truth is that both forms of yoga are good. The one you choose simply depends on where you need help the most. If you are somebody filled with hate and negativity, then try out karma yoga to help yourself act better in life. Then as you begin to feel better in your mind, you won't be critical or skeptical to try out the physical forms of yoga. Best of all, you won't be discouraged by other people either. You will feel what is right in your heart and then proceed.

By the time you are experienced at yoga, you will have enhanced the flexibility and strength in your muscles and joints. This alone is why people feel better after doing yoga for awhile. Some even take it a step further and pursue weight training exercises because their joints and muscles are stronger. Yoga actually becomes a warm up to a regular weight workout for a lot of people because of all the stretching and flexing involved. Of course, you don't have to pursue weight lifting while doing yoga. You could simply take up walking or running exercises as well. Yoga will help you move your legs faster when outside or on the treadmill. Either way, yoga integrates perfectly will all other forms of exercise. But if you only want to do yoga and nothing else, just remember to keep doing yoga as much as you can.

Good luck on your journey into yoga. Keep this book handy and let it be your guide as you progress throughout the beginning stages of yoga

www.ingramcontent.com/pod-product-compliance
Lightning Source LLC
Chambersburg PA
CBHW050840290526
45792CB00001B/467